Better Health Starts Here:
A Doctor's Guide to
Staying Healthy After 40

Better Health Starts Here:
A Doctor's Guide to Staying Healthy After 40

Dr Prabhat Das
MD, PhD, FACP

Better Health with Dr Das Series

Disclaimer
This book is intended solely for educational and informational purposes. It is not meant to replace personal medical advice, diagnosis, or treatment. Although I am a licensed physician, reading this book does not establish a doctor–patient relationship. Each individual's health condition, medical history, and risk factors are unique. Any medical decision should be made in partnership with your own healthcare professional who understands your specific situation.
Medical science is continually advancing. New research and updated guidelines may lead to changes in recommendations over time.

Paperback ISBN: **978-1-971672-16-8**
eBook ISBN: **978-1-971672-17-5**

Typeset in font *Garamond* by *Indica Infomedia*, New Delhi, India
Printed in the United States of America

About the Author

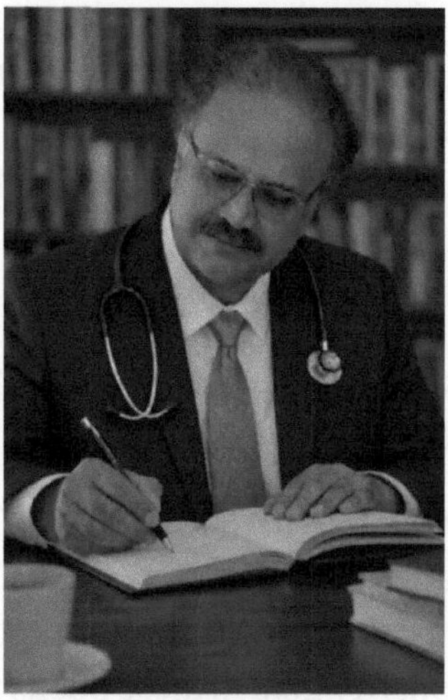

I am **Dr. Prabhat Das, MD, PhD, FACP**. My journey in medicine began in India, and for more than thirty five years I have had the privilege of practicing medicine in the United States. I am trained in **Internal Medicine, Pulmonary Diseases, and Critical Care**, and throughout these decades medicine has been far more than a career for me. It has been a lifelong calling rooted in learning, service, and deep respect for the people who place their trust in their physician.

Over the course of my medical career, I have cared for patients in many different settings. I have seen patients in my office for everyday health concerns, treated people in busy emergency rooms, managed complex illnesses in the hospital, and cared for the most critically ill patients in intensive care units. Thousands of patients have sat across from me during office visits. Many more have depended on careful decisions made during difficult and urgent moments in the hospital and ICU.

But medicine is not only about diagnoses, tests, and treatments. Every day I have listened to patients speak about their worries, their fears, their uncertainty, and often the many questions they hesitate to ask. Those conversations have taught me something profound. People want clear information, honest guidance, and reassurance they can trust. They want to understand their health so they can take better care of themselves and the people they love.

These experiences have shaped how I think about health, illness, prevention, and the deeply human side of healing.

Through the **"Better Health with Dr Das" series**, I hope to reach many individuals I may never meet personally in my office. Many people struggle quietly with health questions and confusing medical information. My goal in these books is simple. I want to explain important medical topics in a clear, practical, and reassuring way so that readers feel informed, confident, and empowered to make better decisions about their health. The information presented in these books is based on reliable scientific knowledge and decades of clinical experience.

If these books bring clarity to someone who feels confused, comfort to someone who feels worried, or practical help to someone trying to improve their health, then this effort will have been deeply worthwhile.

Helping people live healthier, better informed lives continues to be one of the greatest privileges and satisfactions of my professional life.

Table of Contents

About the Author 5

Introduction 11

Chapter 1: Better Health Starts Here: Why This Book May Be One of the Most Important Books You Read 15

Chapter 2: Why I Wrote This Series 23

Chapter 3: Health First 29

Chapter 4: Why Health Matters Even More After 40 37

Chapter 5: Lost in the Noise: Why Modern Health Information Confuses So Many People 43

Chapter 6: Why Reliable Medical Guidance Matters More Than Ever 51

Chapter 7: You Are One Whole Person: Why All Organs and Systems Are Deeply Connected 57

Chapter 8: The True Foundations of Good Health 65

Chapter 9: Food Choices Shape Your Health Every Single Day 73

Chapter 10: Movement: One of the Most Powerful Medicines You Already Have 79

Chapter 11: Sleep, Stress, and Daily Habits: The Quiet Forces That Shape Your Future 85

Chapter 12: When Medicines Help: Why Good Treatment and Good Habits Work Best Together 93

Chapter 13: Prevention and Checkups: The Quiet Protection Most People Undervalue 99

Chapter 14: Do Not Ignore the Signals: Symptoms, Changes, and Warning Signs That Deserve Attention 105

Chapter 15: One Person, Many Health Issues: How to Use This Series to Protect Your Health as a Whole 111

Introduction

Good health is one of life's greatest blessings, yet it is also one of the things people most often take for granted.

As long as the body feels reasonably well, many of us move through life without giving health the attention it deserves. We work hard, stay busy, care for our families, chase goals, and postpone our own needs. We tell ourselves that we will focus on our health when life becomes less demanding. For many people, that time never truly comes. Instead, attention turns toward health only after a troubling symptom appears, a blood test shows an abnormal number, or a doctor raises a concern that can no longer be ignored.

That is how it often begins. Quietly. Gradually. A little weight gain that becomes harder to reverse. Blood pressure that starts to creep upward. Blood sugar that is "a little high." Sleep that is no longer refreshing. Energy that is not what it used to be. A body that seems less forgiving than before.

After 40, these changes begin to matter more. The body still serves us faithfully, but it does not always recover as easily as it once did. Risks that seemed distant when we were younger start to feel more personal. Diabetes, high blood pressure, heart disease, obesity, high cholesterol, poor sleep, and many other problems become more common with age. Some of these conditions develop slowly and silently. A person may feel fine and still have important changes taking place inside the body.

That is one reason health deserves serious attention before illness forces it upon us.

Another reason is the confusion that surrounds health information today. We are living in a time when advice is everywhere. Articles, videos, social media posts, advertisements, influencers, and casual opinions all compete for attention. Some of this information is helpful. Much of it is incomplete, misleading, oversimplified, or driven more by business than by truth. Instead of bringing clarity, it often leaves people more uncertain than before. They hear one recommendation today and another tomorrow. They are told to fear one food, praise another, avoid one medicine, trust another, and somehow make sense of all of it.

This confusion is not a small problem. It affects real people, real decisions, and real health.

Over many years in medical practice, I have seen this clearly. I have cared for patients in offices, hospitals, and critical care settings. I have seen patients come with simple concerns and others come with serious illness. I have listened to their questions, their fears, and the confusion that often sits quietly beneath the surface. Again and again, I have seen the same truth. Most people want to protect their health. They want to make good decisions. They want to avoid disease when possible and manage it wisely when it appears. But many do not have clear, reliable, practical guidance in language they can easily understand.

That is why I wrote this book.

This book was written to give readers a broad, clear, trustworthy understanding of health, especially after 40. It is not a book about one single disease. It is not only about diabetes, or blood pressure, or weight, or cholesterol. It is about the larger picture. It is about how health is built, how it is slowly undermined, and how it can be protected with better understanding and wiser daily choices.

That larger picture matters because the body does not live in separate compartments. For convenience, we often discuss the heart, the kidneys, the brain, blood sugar, blood pressure, cholesterol, sleep, stress, and weight as if they are isolated subjects. In real life, they are deeply connected. Trouble in one area often affects another. Good health in one area supports the rest. A person is never just a diagnosis, a prescription, or a number on a report. A person is a whole human being.

This is also why I created the "**Better Health with Dr Das Series**".

Each book in this series focuses on a particular health topic so that it can be explained clearly and in enough detail. But these books are not meant to stand as rigid, isolated compartments. They are connected by a larger purpose. Together, they are meant to guide the reader as a whole person, not merely as someone with diabetes, or high blood pressure, or a heart problem, or excess weight. Each book adds depth. Each book supports the others. This anchor book serves as the starting point. It helps you understand the foundations of good health and prepares you to use the rest of the series in a more meaningful way.

In the pages ahead, we will discuss some of the most important principles that shape long-term health. We will look at why health should be everyone's number one priority, why it becomes even more valuable with age, why reliable medical guidance matters, and why the body must be understood as a connected whole. We will also explore the true foundations of good health: sound information, healthy eating, regular movement, good sleep, stress control, prevention, checkups, and medicines when they are truly needed.

This book is written especially for adults after 40, but its message is useful at almost any age. Whether you already have a medical condition, want to prevent one, or simply wish to live with more strength, energy, clarity, and independence, this book is for you.

My goal is not merely to provide information. My goal is to reduce confusion, bring perspective, and help you think more clearly about your own health. I want this book to help you become a better-informed, more thoughtful, and more active partner in your own care. Good health is rarely created by one medicine, one lab test, one doctor visit, or one burst of motivation. More often, it is built slowly through understanding, awareness, and repeated daily choices.

That may sound simple, but it is powerful.

Better health does not usually begin with something dramatic. It begins quietly. It begins when a person decides to pay attention. It begins when confusion is replaced by understanding. It begins when small good choices start to happen more often than harmful ones. It begins when we stop waiting for the perfect time and decide that our health is worth protecting now.

That is where this book begins.

That is where better health starts.

Chapter 1

Better Health Starts Here: Why This Book May Be One of the Most Important Books You Read

There are moments in life when we pause and take a quiet look at ourselves.

Not a quick glance in the mirror, but a deeper reflection.

Am I truly taking care of my health?

Am I moving in the right direction?

Or have I been postponing what matters most?

For many people, this moment comes gradually. It may come after a routine checkup when a number is slightly higher than expected. It may come when energy is not what it used to be. It may come after noticing weight gain, poor sleep, or a sense that the body is no longer as forgiving as before.

These are not moments to fear.

They are moments to pay attention.

This book is written for that moment.

Why This Book Deserves Your Attention Now

Most people do not ignore their health intentionally.

Life is full. Responsibilities are many. Work, family, and daily commitments take priority. Health quietly moves to the background. It becomes something we will "take care of later."

But health does not wait.

Changes in the body often begin long before symptoms appear. Blood pressure may rise slowly over the years. Blood sugar may increase little by little. Cholesterol may quietly build up in blood vessels. Weight may increase in small steps that seem harmless at the time.

Because these changes are gradual, they are easy to overlook.

But over time, they begin to matter.

This is why paying attention early is not only wise, it is necessary.

What This Book Will Do for You

This book is not meant to overwhelm you with medical detail.

It is meant to do something more useful.

It is meant to help you:

- Understand your health in a clear and practical way

- See how different aspects of health are connected
- Recognize what truly matters and what does not
- Make better everyday decisions with more confidence

Many people feel uncertain about their health. They hear different opinions, read different advice, and try different approaches. Instead of clarity, they often feel more confused.

This book is written to reduce that confusion.

Why This Is Not Just Another Health Book

There are many books about health.

Some focus on one disease. Others promote one diet, one method, or one idea.

This book takes a different approach.

It does not try to convince you of one narrow solution. Instead, it helps you understand the foundations that support your entire health.

It brings together the key ideas that influence long-term well-being and explains them in a way that connects to real life.

Rather than offering isolated advice, it gives you a broader perspective.

And that perspective is what allows better decisions.

Why Understanding Comes Before Lasting Change

Many people try to improve their health by making sudden

changes.

They start a strict diet. They begin exercising intensely. They follow advice they have heard without fully understanding it.

Some of these efforts work for a short time.

Many do not last.

Without understanding, it is difficult to remain consistent.

When you understand:

- Why a change matters
- How it affects your body
- What results to expect

you are more likely to stay with it.

Understanding builds confidence.

Confidence supports consistency.

Consistency leads to real results.

The Power of Small, Steady Choices

There is a common belief that big changes lead to big results.

In health, this is often not true.

Health is usually built through small, steady choices made every day:

- What you eat
- How much you move

- How well you sleep
- How you manage stress
- Whether you take your medicines properly
- Whether you go for regular checkups

These choices may seem minor on any given day.

But over months and years, they shape your future.

Many people look for quick results. In reality, steady and consistent habits are far more powerful than short bursts of effort.

How This Book Prepares You for the Rest of the Series

This book is the beginning of a larger journey.

In the rest of this series, we will look more closely at specific conditions such as obesity, diabetes, high blood pressure, cholesterol, and other common health concerns.

But before going into those details, it is important to understand the bigger picture.

This book provides that foundation.

When you read the other books after this one, you will:

- Understand them more clearly
- See how they are connected
- Apply their guidance more effectively

Think of this book as a map.

The other books will help you explore different parts of that map in greater depth.

Chapter Summary

- Health changes often begin quietly and gradually.
- Waiting for symptoms may delay important action.
- Understanding your health is the first step toward improvement.
- Small daily choices shape long-term outcomes.
- This book provides the foundation for the entire series.

Action Plan

- Take a few quiet minutes to reflect on your current health.
- Ask yourself honestly: *Have I been postponing my health?*
- Identify one area where you can improve.
- Start with one small, realistic step this week.
- Read this book thoughtfully, with attention and intention.

Bridge to Chapter 2

Now that you understand what this book is meant to do, an important question remains.

Why was this series written in the first place?

What need does it address?

And how can it help you in ways that other sources may not?

Let us explore that next.

Chapter 2

Why I Wrote This Series: Lessons from Years of Caring for Patients

Over the years, I have had the privilege of caring for patients in many different settings. I have seen people come in for routine visits, I have treated those who were unwell but stable, and I have also taken care of patients in serious and critical conditions.

Through all these experiences, one pattern has remained clear.

Most people genuinely want to stay healthy. They want to make good decisions. They want to avoid disease if possible and manage it wisely when it appears.

But many are unsure how to do that.

This series was written to bridge that gap.

What Years of Practice Have Quietly Taught Me

In day-to-day practice, I have seen the same story repeat itself.

A patient comes in with a condition that has been developing for years. High blood pressure that was never monitored regularly. Blood sugar that remained slightly elevated but was not taken seriously. Gradual weight gain that slowly became significant. Cholesterol levels that stayed high without consistent follow-up.

In many cases, these problems did not appear suddenly.

They developed quietly, over time.

What is most striking is that many of these conditions could have been better controlled, or even delayed, with earlier awareness and simple, steady steps.

Why Many People Remain Confused About Their Health

This confusion is not due to lack of interest.

Most people care deeply about their health. But they face several challenges:

- Medical visits are often brief
- A lot of information is shared in a short time
- Medical terms can be difficult to understand
- Questions often arise after the visit is over

As a result, many patients leave with partial understanding.

They may:

- Forget important details
- Misinterpret instructions

- Feel uncertain about what to do next

This uncertainty can lead to hesitation, delay, or inconsistent care.

The Questions Patients Often Carry but Do Not Ask

Over time, I have realized that many patients carry important questions that are not always expressed.

They may wonder:

- How serious is my condition?
- Do I really need this medicine?
- Can I control this without medication?
- What happens if I delay treatment?
- What should I change in my daily life?

These are not small questions.

They deserve clear, thoughtful answers.

When these questions remain unanswered, people often turn to other sources, which may not always be reliable.

Why Clear, Practical Medical Explanation Is So Important

Medical science has advanced tremendously.

We understand many diseases better than ever before. We have effective treatments and preventive strategies.

But knowledge is only useful when it is understood.

Too often, explanations are either:

- Too technical
- Too brief
- Too disconnected from real-life concerns

What people need is something different.

They need:

- Clear language
- Practical guidance
- Balanced explanation
- Advice that fits real life

That is what I have tried to provide in this series.

Why I Chose to Write a Series, Not Just One Book

Health cannot be fully explained in a single book.

At the same time, it should not be reduced to a few general statements.

That is why I chose to write a series.

Each book focuses on one important area so it can be explained clearly and in enough depth. At the same time, all the books are connected.

This approach allows:

- Clarity without oversimplification

- Depth without confusion
- Practical guidance without losing the bigger picture

What I Hope This Series Will Do for You

My goal is not only to give you information.

My goal is to help you:

- Understand your health more clearly
- Feel less confused and less anxious
- Make better everyday decisions
- Ask better questions during medical visits
- Take a more active role in your own care

I also want you to feel more confident.

Health does not have to feel overwhelming.

With the right understanding, it becomes more manageable.

Chapter Summary

- Many common health problems develop slowly over time.
- Patients often feel confused because they do not receive enough clear explanation.
- Important questions often remain unasked and unanswered.
- Clear, practical, and reliable medical guidance is needed.

- This series is designed to provide that guidance in a connected and meaningful way.

Action Plan

- Reflect on your own health journey so far.
- Ask yourself: *What do I still not fully understand about my health?*
- Write down two or three important questions you have.
- Decide to become more engaged and informed about your health.
- Use this series as a guide, not just as reading material.

Bridge to Chapter 3

Now that you understand why this series was written, the next question becomes even more important.

Why should health be treated as the highest priority in your life?

What really changes when health begins to decline?

Let us explore that next.

Chapter 3

Health First

Why Nothing Matters More When Health Begins to Slip

There is a quiet truth most of us recognize, yet often overlook.

As long as we feel reasonably well, we move through life without thinking much about our health. We work, plan, travel, enjoy time with family, and take care of daily responsibilities. Health remains in the background, doing its job silently.

Then, something changes.

It may be a number on a report. It may be a new symptom. It may be a feeling that the body is not as strong or dependable as before.

And suddenly, health moves to the center of everything.

This chapter is about understanding that truth before it is forced upon us.

Why Health Is the Foundation of Everything You Do

Every part of your life rests on your health.

Your ability to:

- Work and stay productive
- Think clearly and make decisions
- Enjoy time with family and friends
- Travel, move, and remain active
- Sleep well and wake with energy

all depend on how well your body and mind are functioning.

When health is strong, life feels normal.

When health weakens, even simple things can become difficult.

Health is not just one part of life. It supports every part of life.

How Illness Quietly Changes Daily Life

When health begins to decline, the change is often gradual.

You may notice:

- Less energy than before
- Reduced stamina
- More frequent discomfort
- Greater dependence on medicines
- Increased worry about symptoms

Activities that once felt effortless may require more effort.

The focus of life slowly shifts:

- From planning to managing
- From enjoying to adjusting
- From freedom to limitation

This change can be subtle at first, but over time it becomes deeply felt.

Why We Often Delay Taking Health Seriously

Many people do not neglect their health out of carelessness.

They delay for understandable reasons:

- Busy schedules
- Family and work responsibilities
- The feeling that "nothing serious is wrong"
- The habit of postponing checkups or changes

Sometimes there is also a quiet hope that small problems will resolve on their own.

Unfortunately, many health conditions do not improve without attention.

They often progress quietly.

The Real Cost of Neglecting Health

Neglecting health has consequences that go beyond the body.

It can affect:

- Emotional well-being
- Confidence and independence
- Relationships with family
- Financial stability

Medical care may become more complex. Treatment may become more demanding. Daily life may require more adjustments.

What could have been managed early with simple steps may later require more intensive care.

This is the cost of delay.

Why Taking Care of Your Health Is Not Selfish

Some people feel that focusing on their own health is selfish.

In reality, it is responsible.

When you take care of your health:

- You remain more independent
- You are better able to support your family
- You reduce the burden on others
- You maintain your ability to live fully

Your health affects not only you, but those around you.

Protecting it is a wise and thoughtful choice.

Why Now Is the Right Time to Act

There is no perfect moment to begin taking health seriously.

But there is always a right moment.

That moment is now.

You do not need to wait for:

- A diagnosis
- A symptom
- A crisis

The earlier you begin, the more options you have and the better your long-term outcomes can be.

Even small changes, started today, can lead to meaningful results over time.

Chapter Summary

- Health supports every important aspect of life.
- Illness can gradually change daily living and independence.
- Many people delay attention to health until problems become significant.
- Neglecting health has physical, emotional, and practical costs.
- Taking care of your health is wise, necessary, and benefits both you and your family.

WHY HEALTH IS MOST IMPORTANT

How Prioritizing Your Health Improves Every Part of Your Life

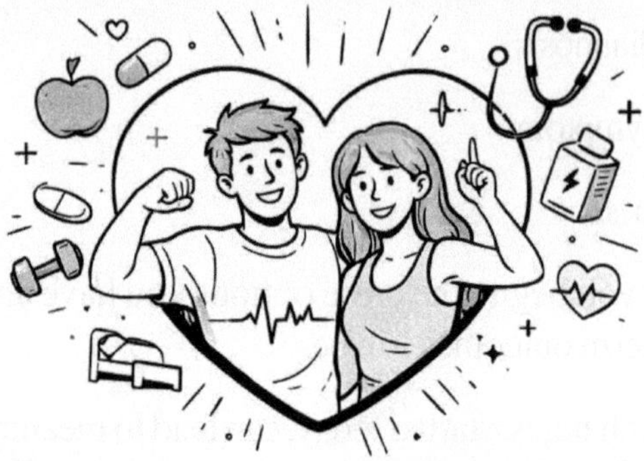

MORE ENERGY
Boosts your vitality and stamina.

BETTER MOOD
Elevates your happiness and reduces stress.

LONGEVITY
Supports a longer, healthın life.

SHARPER MIND
Improves focus, memory, and mental clarity.

MORE PRODUCTIVE
Increases your productivity and performance.

HAPPIER RELATIONSHIPS
Enhances connection with loved ones.

HOW TO PRIORITIZE YOUR HEALTH

- ☑ Eat a balanced, nutritious diet.
- ☑ Exercise regularly, stay active.
- ☑ Get enough quality sleep.
- ☑ Manage stress and relax.

Action Plan

- Take a few quiet minutes to reflect on your current health.
- Ask yourself: *Am I giving my health the attention it deserves?*
- Identify one area where you have been delaying action.
- Take one practical step this week, such as scheduling a checkup or improving a daily habit.
- Remind yourself that small steps today can prevent larger problems later.

Bridge to Chapter 4

If health matters at every stage of life, it becomes even more valuable as we grow older.

What changes in the body after 40?

Why do certain health risks increase?

Let us explore that next.

Chapter 4

Why Health Matters Even More After 40

There is a moment in life, often somewhere in our forties, when we begin to notice subtle changes in ourselves.

Nothing dramatic. Nothing alarming at first.

Just small shifts.

Energy is not quite the same. Weight seems easier to gain and harder to lose. Sleep may become lighter. Recovery after physical effort takes a little longer. A routine checkup shows numbers that are "slightly higher" than before.

These changes are not signs of failure.

They are signals of transition.

After 40, the body is still strong and capable, but it begins to ask for more attention.

What Begins to Change in the Body After 40

As we move into midlife, several gradual changes take place.

Metabolism may slow down. Muscle mass may begin to decrease. Blood vessels may lose some of their flexibility. Hormonal patterns may shift. The body's ability to recover quickly may be reduced.

These changes are usually slow and subtle.

But over time, they can influence:

- Weight
- Blood pressure
- Blood sugar
- Cholesterol
- Energy level
- Sleep quality

Understanding these changes is not meant to create worry. It is meant to create awareness.

Why Certain Health Conditions Become More Common

With age, the likelihood of certain conditions increases.

These include:

- High blood pressure
- Diabetes
- High cholesterol

- Obesity
- Heart disease
- Sleep-related problems

These conditions often do not begin suddenly.

They develop quietly, over years.

Many people are surprised when they are diagnosed because they felt normal for a long time.

This is why awareness becomes more important than ever.

Why Feeling Well May Not Always Mean Being Well

One of the most important lessons in health is simple, but not always obvious.

You can feel well and still have important changes taking place in your body.

High blood pressure may not cause symptoms.

High cholesterol may not be felt.

Early diabetes may go unnoticed.

Because there is no immediate discomfort, these problems can remain hidden.

During this time, silent damage may slowly develop.

This is why relying only on how you feel is not enough.

The Growing Importance of Prevention

As we get older, prevention becomes more valuable.

When we are younger, the body often compensates for unhealthy habits. It recovers more easily.

With time, this ability decreases.

Simple steps such as:

- Eating more carefully
- Staying physically active
- Maintaining a healthy weight
- Monitoring key health indicators
- Managing stress
- Getting adequate sleep

can make a significant difference.

Prevention is not about perfection. It is about reducing risk and protecting the future.

Why Strength, Energy, and Independence Matter So Much

Health is not only about avoiding disease.

It is about preserving the ability to live well.

Strength allows you to move freely.

Energy allows you to stay engaged in life.

Independence allows you to make your own choices.

These are deeply valuable.

Protecting them should be one of the main goals of good health after 40.

How the Years Ahead Can Still Be Healthy and Fulfilling

Aging is not only about decline.

It can also be a time of better awareness and wiser decisions.

Many people become healthier after 40 because they begin to:

- Pay more attention to their bodies
- Make more thoughtful choices
- Seek reliable guidance
- Value their health more deeply

With the right approach, the years ahead can be active, meaningful, and fulfilling.

Chapter Summary

- The body undergoes gradual changes after 40.
- Many health conditions become more common with age.
- Feeling well does not always mean everything is normal.
- Prevention becomes more important over time.
- Health after 40 is about maintaining strength, energy, and independence.

Action Plan

- Reflect on changes you have noticed in your body over recent years.
- Do not ignore gradual shifts in weight, energy, or stamina.
- Schedule regular checkups if you have been postponing them.
- Focus on prevention rather than waiting for symptoms.
- Begin making small, consistent improvements in your daily habits.

Bridge to Chapter 5

As people become more aware of their health, they often begin to search for information.

They read articles, watch videos, and listen to advice from many different sources.

But instead of clarity, they often find confusion.

Why does this happen?

Let us explore that next.

Chapter 5

Lost in the Noise: Why Modern Health Information Confuses So Many People

We are living in a time when information is everywhere.

If you have a question about your health, you can find an answer within seconds. You can read articles, watch videos, listen to podcasts, and scroll through endless opinions.

At first, this feels empowering.

But very often, it leads to something else.

Confusion.

The Flood of Health Information in Everyday Life

Health advice now comes from many directions:

- Internet articles and websites

- Social media platforms
- Videos, podcasts, and online discussions
- Advertisements and product promotions
- Friends, family, and casual conversations

Each source may offer a different message.

One recommends a certain diet. Another warns against it. One praises a supplement. Another questions its safety. One promotes a new trend. Another dismisses it.

Instead of clarity, many people are left wondering what to believe.

Why More Information Does Not Always Mean Better Understanding

Information alone is not enough.

Understanding requires:

- Accuracy
- Context
- Balance
- Relevance to your individual situation

Without these, even correct information can be misused.

For example:

A diet that works well for one person may not be suitable for another. A treatment that is helpful in one situation may not be appropriate in another.

Without context, information can mislead rather than guide.

The Common Traps of Misleading Health Advice

Not all health information is created with the same level of care or responsibility.

Some common problems include:

- **Oversimplification**

  Complex medical issues are reduced to simple slogans or quick solutions.

- **Exaggeration**

  Benefits are overstated while risks are ignored.

- **Selective presentation**

  Only part of the truth is shown, leaving out important details.

- **Commercial influence**

  Advice may be shaped by the goal of selling a product.

- **One-size-fits-all thinking**

  The same advice is applied to everyone without considering individual differences.

These patterns can make unreliable information appear convincing.

How Confusion Leads to Delay and Poor Decisions

Confusion is not harmless.

When people are unsure:

- They may delay seeking proper care
- They may try ineffective or unsafe remedies
- They may stop necessary treatment
- They may feel anxious and overwhelmed

Sometimes, important time is lost.

Sometimes, simple problems become more complicated.

Clarity is not just helpful. It is protective.

Why Non-Medical Advice Often Sounds Convincing

Many sources of health advice present their ideas with great confidence.

They may use:

- Personal stories
- Testimonials
- Emotional language
- Repetition of strong claims

These methods can make the message feel trustworthy.

But confidence is not the same as accuracy.

It is important to remember this distinction.

How to Become a More Careful Judge of Health Information

In today's world, learning how to evaluate information is an essential skill.

A few simple habits can help:

- Ask who is providing the information
- Consider whether they have medical training
- Look for balanced explanations rather than extreme claims
- Be cautious about quick fixes and guaranteed results
- Compare information from more than one reliable source

Over time, these habits can reduce confusion and improve your decisions.

Chapter Summary

- Health information is widely available but not always reliable.
- More information does not automatically lead to better understanding.
- Misleading advice can appear convincing and influence decisions.
- Confusion can delay proper care and lead to poor choices.
- Learning to evaluate information is an important part of protecting your health.

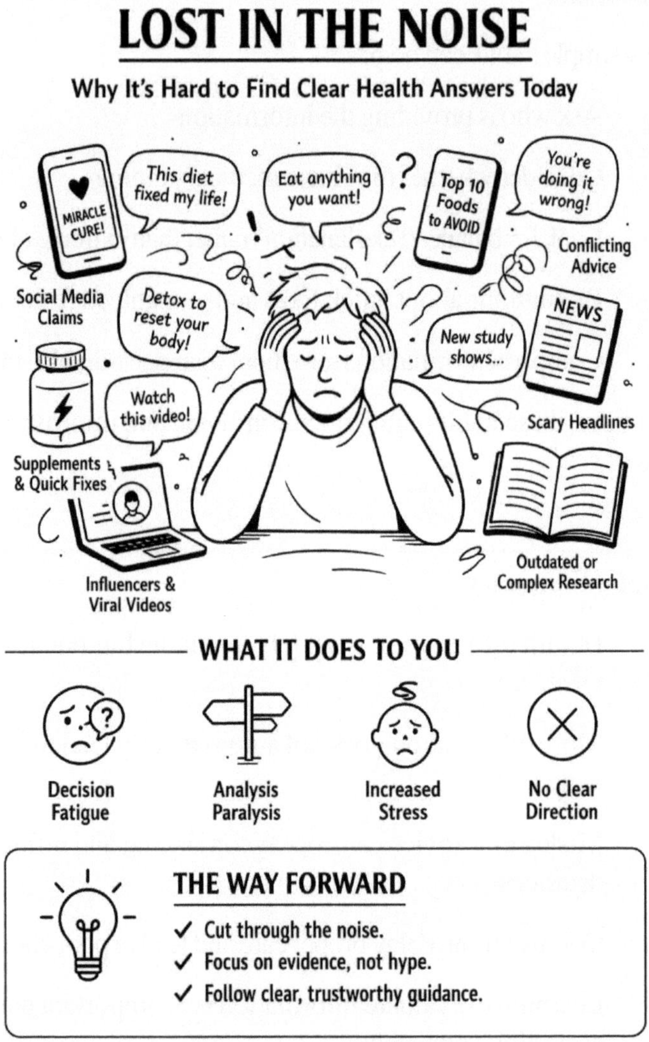
LOST IN THE NOISE
Why It's Hard to Find Clear Health Answers Today
MIRACLE CURE!
This diet fixed my life!
Eat anything you want!
Top 10 Foods to AVOID
You're doing it wrong!
Conflicting Advice
Social Media Claims
Detox to reset your body!
NEWS
New study shows...
Watch this video!
Scary Headlines
Supplements & Quick Fixes
Influencers & Viral Videos
Outdated or Complex Research
WHAT IT DOES TO YOU
Decision Fatigue
Analysis Paralysis
Increased Stress
No Clear Direction
THE WAY FORWARD
✓ Cut through the noise.
✓ Focus on evidence, not hype.
✓ Follow clear, trustworthy guidance.

Action Plan

- Review where you usually get your health information.
- Identify any sources that may not be reliable.
- Be cautious about dramatic claims and quick solutions.
- Begin to rely more on medically sound, credible sources.
- Pause and think before acting on new advice.

Bridge to Chapter 6

If confusion is one of the biggest challenges in modern health, then reliable guidance becomes even more valuable.

Where should you turn for trustworthy advice?

What makes medical guidance dependable?

Let us explore that next.

Chapter 6

Why Reliable Medical Guidance Matters More Than Ever

In a world full of advice, opinions, and endless information, one question becomes very important.

Whom should you trust when it comes to your health?

This question may seem simple, but the answer can shape your decisions, your treatment, and your long-term well-being.

Reliable guidance does more than provide information.

It gives direction.

It helps you understand what matters, what does not, and what you should do next.

What Makes Doctor-Guided Information More Dependable

Medical knowledge is not built overnight.

It comes from years of structured learning, careful training, and ongoing experience.

Doctors spend years understanding:

- How the body functions
- How diseases develop
- How different conditions are diagnosed
- How treatments affect different individuals

Beyond knowledge, there is experience.

Seeing many patients over time allows a physician to recognize patterns, understand variations, and make balanced decisions.

Doctor-guided information is based on both science and real-life experience.

Why Health Decisions Must Fit the Whole Person

No two individuals are exactly the same.

A recommendation that works well for one person may not be suitable for another.

Health decisions depend on several factors:

- Age
- Existing medical conditions
- Medications already in use
- Family history
- Lifestyle

- Personal risk

Good medical guidance takes all of these into account.

It does not offer identical answers for everyone.

The Difference Between Medical Judgment and Casual Opinion

There is a clear difference between informed medical judgment and casual opinion.

Medical judgment is based on:

- Scientific evidence
- Clinical experience
- Understanding of benefits and risks

Casual opinion may be based on:

- Personal experience
- Partial information
- Popular trends

Both may sound convincing.

But they are not equal.

When it comes to your health, the quality of advice matters greatly.

Why Good Guidance Is Balanced, Not Extreme

Reliable medical advice avoids extremes.

It does not:

- Promise instant cures
- Ignore possible risks
- Simplify complex problems too much

Instead, it aims to:

- Present both benefits and limitations
- Acknowledge uncertainty when it exists
- Offer practical and realistic recommendations

This balanced approach helps you make thoughtful decisions.

How Reliable Information Reduces Fear and Improves Action

Uncertainty often leads to anxiety.

When people do not understand their condition or treatment, they may feel worried or hesitant.

Clear and reliable information can:

- Reduce unnecessary fear
- Build confidence
- Improve adherence to treatment
- Encourage timely action

Understanding gives a sense of control.

How to Use Books, Doctors, and Credible Sources Together

Health information works best when it is used wisely.

Books like this one can:

- Provide a broader understanding
- Explain concepts in detail
- Help you prepare better questions

Your doctor can:

- Apply that knowledge to your individual situation
- Offer personalized recommendations
- Monitor your progress

Together, these sources create a stronger foundation for good decisions.

Chapter Summary

- Reliable medical guidance is essential in a world full of information.
- Doctor-guided advice is based on training, evidence, and experience.
- Health decisions must consider the whole person.
- Balanced guidance is more useful than extreme claims.
- Understanding reduces fear and improves decision-making.

Action Plan

- Choose to rely on credible, medically sound sources.
- Avoid making important decisions based on casual opinions.
- Prepare questions before your medical visits.
- Use reading as a tool to deepen understanding, not replace care.
- Work in partnership with your doctor.

Bridge to Chapter 7

Good medical guidance always looks at the person as a whole.

It does not treat the heart, kidneys, brain, or metabolism as separate, unrelated parts.

Why is this important?

How are different systems in the body connected?

Let us explore that next.

Chapter 7

You Are One Whole Person: Why All Organs and Systems Are Deeply Connected

One of the most important truths in medicine is also one of the easiest to overlook.

You are not a collection of separate organs.

You are one whole, connected system.

For the sake of learning, we often divide the body into parts. We talk about the heart, lungs, kidneys, brain, blood sugar, blood pressure, and cholesterol as if they exist independently.

But in real life, nothing in the body works in isolation.

Understanding this can change how you think about your health in a deeper and more meaningful way.

Why the Body Works as One Integrated System

Every organ in the body depends on others.

The heart pumps blood, but it relies on healthy blood vessels.

The brain directs functions, but it depends on oxygen and proper circulation.

The kidneys filter waste, but they depend on steady blood flow.

Even systems that seem unrelated are closely linked.

Blood carries oxygen, nutrients, hormones, and signals throughout the body. These connections allow different organs to communicate and function together.

This coordination is constant.

How One Problem Can Affect Many Areas of the Body

When one part of the body is affected, the effects often extend beyond that area.

For example:

- High blood pressure can strain the heart and damage the kidneys
- Diabetes can affect blood vessels, nerves, eyes, and kidneys
- Obesity can influence joints, metabolism, breathing, and circulation
- Poor sleep can affect energy, blood pressure, and blood sugar

These are not isolated problems.

They are connected patterns.

That is why a single issue should never be viewed in isolation.

Why Common Health Conditions Often Occur Together

Many common conditions seen after 40 tend to occur together.

These include:

- Obesity
- Diabetes
- High blood pressure
- High cholesterol
- Heart disease

They share common underlying factors such as:

- Diet
- Physical inactivity
- Stress
- Metabolic changes
- Genetic influences

Improving one area often helps others.

Ignoring one area can worsen several others.

Why Mental and Emotional Health Also Matter

Health is not only physical.

Mental and emotional well-being have a strong influence on the body.

Stress, anxiety, and poor sleep can:

- Raise blood pressure
- Affect appetite and eating patterns
- Reduce motivation for healthy habits
- Influence energy and mood

At the same time, physical illness can affect emotional well-being.

The connection works both ways.

Why Focusing on One Problem Alone Is Not Enough

Sometimes people try to manage one condition without considering the bigger picture.

For example:

- Treating blood pressure without addressing weight or stress
- Managing blood sugar without improving diet or activity
- Taking medication but neglecting daily habits

These approaches may help partially, but they are often incomplete.

A broader, more integrated approach leads to better results.

Why This Series Focuses on the Whole Person

In this book series, each condition is discussed separately for clarity.

But this separation is only for understanding.

In real life, these conditions are interconnected.

You are not just:

- A diagnosis
- A number on a lab report
- A prescription

You are a whole person.

The goal of this series is to help you understand each part while always keeping the whole in mind.

Chapter Summary

- The body functions as an interconnected system.
- Problems in one area often affect other areas.
- Many common conditions are closely linked.
- Mental and emotional health influence physical health.
- A whole-person approach leads to better understanding and outcomes.

Health as a Connected System

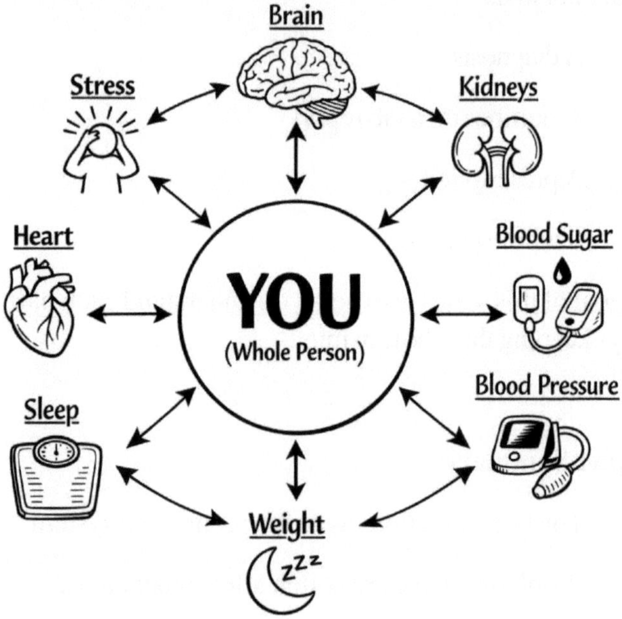

All systems are connected. One problem affects many others.

Action Plan

- Begin thinking of your health as a connected system.
- Reflect on how different aspects of your health may be influencing each other.
- Avoid focusing on only one issue while ignoring others.
- Make changes that can benefit multiple areas of health.
- Discuss your overall health, not just individual symptoms, during medical visits.

Bridge to Chapter 8

Now that you understand how deeply connected the body is, the next step is to look at what supports this entire system.

What are the key foundations that keep the body healthy over time?

Let us explore those foundations next.

Chapter 8

The True Foundations of Good Health

What Really Keeps You Well Over Time

When people think about health, they often think about diseases.

They think about diabetes, high blood pressure, heart disease, or cholesterol. They think about tests, medicines, and doctor visits.

But long before disease develops, there are deeper forces quietly shaping your health every single day.

These are the foundations of health.

If these foundations are strong, your body is better protected.

If they are weak, problems slowly begin to develop.

Understanding these foundations is one of the most important steps toward lasting health.

What the Foundations of Health Really Are

Good health does not depend on one single factor.

It rests on several key pillars:

- What you eat
- How much you move
- How well you sleep
- How you handle stress
- Whether you receive reliable information
- Whether you seek timely medical care

These may seem simple, but they are powerful.

Each of these influences multiple systems in the body. Together, they determine the direction your health takes over time.

Why Health Is Built by Routine, Not Rescue

Many people pay attention to health only when a problem appears.

At that point, they try to "fix" it quickly.

But health is rarely repaired overnight.

It is built gradually, through daily habits.

For example:

- Eating reasonably well most days is more important than eating perfectly for a short time
- Moving regularly matters more than exercising intensely

once in a while

- Sleeping consistently well is more valuable than occasional long rest

Routine is what shapes long-term health.

Why Prevention Is More Powerful Than Treatment

Treating disease is important.

But preventing disease is often simpler and more effective.

Once a condition develops, it may require:

- Long-term medication
- Regular monitoring
- Lifestyle adjustments

Prevention often involves:

- Better daily habits
- Regular checkups
- Early attention to small changes

It reduces risk before damage occurs.

Why No Single Habit Can Protect Your Health Alone

Some people focus only on one aspect of health.

They may:

- Exercise regularly but eat poorly
- Eat well but remain inactive
- Take medicines but neglect sleep and stress

No single habit is enough.

The body responds best when multiple areas are addressed together.

Balance is essential.

How Strong Foundations Protect the Whole Body

One of the most encouraging truths about health is this:

Improving one habit often benefits several areas at once.

For example:

- Better diet can improve weight, blood sugar, blood pressure, and cholesterol
- Regular movement can improve heart health, strength, and mood
- Good sleep can improve energy, focus, and metabolic balance

These benefits are interconnected.

That is why strengthening your foundations has wide-reaching effects.

How Weak Foundations Quietly Lead to Disease

When healthy habits are neglected, the effects may not be immediate.

But over time:

- Poor diet may lead to weight gain and metabolic problems
- Inactivity may reduce strength and increase disease risk
- Poor sleep may affect energy, mood, and hormones
- Chronic stress may influence multiple body systems

These changes often develop slowly and silently.

By the time they become noticeable, they may already be established.

Chapter Summary

- Good health is built on a few key foundations.
- Daily habits matter more than occasional efforts.
- Prevention is often more effective than treatment.
- No single habit can protect health alone.
- Strong foundations benefit multiple systems in the body.

Action Plan

- Review the main foundations of your health honestly.
- Ask yourself:

FOUNDATION OF GOOD HEALTH

KEY ELEMENTS

BALANCED NUTRITION

Consumes a variety of nutritious foods.

REGULAR EXERCISE

Engages in physical activity consistently.

ADEQUATE SLEEP

Gets sufficient and restful sleep.

STRESS MANAGEMENT

Maintains mental well-being.

PREVENTIVE CARE

Attends regular health check-ups.

    - Am I eating well most days?
    - Am I moving regularly?
    - Am I sleeping adequately?
    - Am I managing stress effectively?
- Identify one area that needs improvement.
- Begin with one small, sustainable change.
- Focus on consistency rather than perfection.

Bridge to Chapter 9

Among all the foundations of health, one stands out because it affects you multiple times every day.

That foundation is food.

What you eat, how you eat, and how often you eat all play a major role in shaping your health.

Let us explore that next.

Chapter 9

Food Choices Shape Your Health Every Single Day

Food is one of the few things in life that we interact with every day, often several times a day.

It is not just nourishment.

It is information for your body.

Every meal you eat sends signals. It influences your metabolism, your energy, your hormones, and over time, your risk for disease.

Because it is so routine, it is easy to overlook its importance.

But few factors shape long-term health as powerfully as food.

Why Food Is More Than Calories

Many people think of food mainly in terms of calories.

Calories matter, but they are only part of the story.

Food also provides:

- Nutrients that support body function
- Building blocks for muscles and tissues
- Signals that influence metabolism and hormones

The type of food you eat affects how your body responds.

For example:

- Some foods raise blood sugar quickly
- Some keep energy steady
- Some increase inflammation
- Some support long-term health

Understanding food beyond calories helps you make better choices.

How Modern Eating Patterns Quietly Harm Health

Over time, eating habits have changed in ways that are not always helpful.

Many people now rely more on:

- Processed and packaged foods
- Meals high in sugar, salt, and unhealthy fats
- Large portion sizes
- Frequent snacking without true hunger

These patterns can gradually lead to:

- Weight gain
- Increased blood sugar
- Higher blood pressure
- Unhealthy cholesterol levels

Because these changes develop slowly, they are easy to ignore until problems appear.

Why Healthy Eating Does Not Require Extreme Diets

There is a common belief that improving diet requires strict rules or major restrictions.

In reality, most people do better with a simpler approach.

Healthy eating does not mean:

- Eliminating all favorite foods
- Following complicated plans
- Making sudden, extreme changes

It usually means:

- Choosing more natural, whole foods
- Reducing excess sugar, salt, and processed items
- Eating balanced meals
- Practicing moderation

Simplicity makes habits easier to maintain.

Common Mistakes That Make Healthy Eating Difficult

Many people try to improve their diet but struggle to sustain it.

Some common mistakes include:

- Starting very strict diets that are difficult to maintain
- Expecting quick results
- Following trends without understanding them
- Skipping meals and overeating later
- Ignoring portion sizes

These patterns often lead to cycles of effort and frustration.

The Link Between Food and Long-Term Health

Food plays a major role in preventing many common conditions.

A balanced diet can help:

- Maintain a healthy weight
- Improve blood sugar control
- Lower blood pressure
- Reduce cholesterol
- Support heart and brain health

On the other hand, poor eating habits can increase the risk of these conditions over time.

The effects may be gradual, but they are significant.

Building a Practical and Sustainable Way of Eating

The goal is not perfection.

The goal is consistency.

A practical approach may include:

- Eating regular meals instead of constant snacking
- Including vegetables, fruits, and whole foods more often
- Reducing sugary drinks and processed snacks
- Being mindful of portion sizes
- Allowing flexibility without guilt

Healthy eating should feel realistic, not restrictive.

Chapter Summary

- Food affects many aspects of health every day.
- It is more than calories and influences metabolism and long-term risk.
- Modern eating patterns often contribute to health problems.
- Healthy eating does not require extreme diets.
- Sustainable habits are more important than temporary efforts.

Action Plan

- Review your current eating habits honestly.
- Identify one pattern that may be harming your health.
- Reduce or replace one unhealthy food habit this week.
- Focus on balance rather than strict rules.
- Aim for steady, long-term improvement.

Bridge to Chapter 10

Food is a powerful foundation of health, but it is only part of the picture.

The body is designed to move.

When movement is reduced, many systems begin to suffer.

Let us now look at how movement shapes your health.

Chapter 10

Movement: One of the Most Powerful Medicines You Already Have

The human body is built for movement.

Yet, in modern life, movement has quietly disappeared from many of our daily routines. We sit for long hours at work, during travel, and even during leisure time. What was once a naturally active life has gradually become more sedentary.

This change has not been harmless.

It has affected our strength, our energy, and our long-term health.

The good news is simple and encouraging.

Movement is one of the most powerful tools you have to improve your health, and it is already within your reach.

Why the Body Needs Movement to Stay Healthy

Every system in the body depends on regular movement.

When you move:

- Muscles stay strong
- Joints remain flexible
- Blood circulates more efficiently
- The heart becomes more effective
- Metabolism stays active

Movement also helps regulate:

- Blood sugar
- Blood pressure
- Cholesterol

It supports mental well-being by improving mood and reducing stress.

The body functions best when it is used regularly.

What Happens When Movement Is Missing

When activity decreases, the body begins to adapt in less helpful ways.

A sedentary lifestyle can lead to:

- Muscle weakness
- Reduced flexibility

- Weight gain
- Poor stamina
- Increased risk of diabetes, heart disease, and other conditions

These changes often happen slowly.

Because they are gradual, they may not be noticed until they begin to interfere with daily life.

Exercise and Everyday Movement: Both Matter

Many people think of physical activity only as formal exercise.

While structured exercise is important, everyday movement also plays a key role.

Exercise may include:

- Walking for fitness
- Strength training
- Cycling, swimming, or similar activities

Everyday movement includes:

- Walking around the home or workplace
- Climbing stairs
- Doing household tasks
- Standing and moving during the day

Both types of movement contribute to better health.

Even small increases in activity can make a meaningful difference.

The Benefits of Different Types of Movement

Different forms of movement provide different benefits.

- **Aerobic activity**

  Improves heart health, circulation, and stamina

- **Strength training**

  Helps maintain muscle mass and supports joints

- **Flexibility exercises**

  Reduce stiffness and improve mobility

- **Balance exercises**

  Help prevent falls and improve stability

A balanced approach that includes different types of movement is ideal.

Why Starting Small Leads to Lasting Success

Many people delay becoming active because they feel they need a perfect plan.

In reality, simple beginnings are often more effective.

You do not need:

- A gym membership
- Expensive equipment

- A complicated routine

You can begin with:

- Short daily walks
- Light stretching
- Gradual increases in activity

Starting small reduces the risk of injury and makes it easier to stay consistent.

Making Movement a Natural Part of Daily Life

The key to long-term benefit is consistency.

Movement becomes sustainable when it is part of your routine.

Some practical ways include:

- Setting a regular time for walking
- Taking short movement breaks during the day
- Choosing stairs instead of elevators when possible
- Incorporating activity into daily tasks

Over time, these habits become natural.

Chapter Summary

- Movement is essential for maintaining health.
- A sedentary lifestyle can gradually harm the body.

- Both exercise and everyday movement are important.
- Different types of activity provide different benefits.
- Starting small and staying consistent leads to lasting improvement.

Action Plan

- Assess how much time you spend sitting each day.
- Add one simple movement habit, such as a daily walk.
- Break long periods of sitting with short activity.
- Choose activities you enjoy and can maintain.
- Focus on consistency rather than intensity.

Bridge to Chapter 11

Even with good nutrition and regular movement, health can still be affected by factors that are less visible.

Sleep, stress, and daily habits quietly shape how the body functions.

Let us explore these important influences next.

Chapter 11

Sleep, Stress, and Daily Habits: The Quiet Forces That Shape Your Future

Some of the most powerful influences on your health are not dramatic.

They do not appear suddenly. They do not always draw attention.

They work quietly, in the background, shaping how you feel and how your body functions every single day.

These influences are:

- How well you sleep
- How much stress you carry
- How your daily habits are structured

Over time, they can strengthen your health or slowly weaken it.

Why Sleep Is Essential for Health

Sleep is not just rest. It is active recovery.

During sleep, the body:

- Repairs tissues
- Regulates hormones
- Strengthens the immune system
- Processes memory and learning

Good sleep supports:

- Energy and alertness
- Emotional balance
- Healthy metabolism

Poor sleep can lead to:

- Fatigue
- Reduced concentration
- Increased appetite
- Higher blood pressure
- Poor blood sugar control

Many people underestimate the importance of consistent, restful sleep.

How Stress Affects the Body Over Time

Stress is a natural part of life.

In small amounts, it can be helpful. It can increase focus and help you respond to challenges.

But when stress becomes constant, it begins to affect the body.

Chronic stress can:

- Raise blood pressure
- Disrupt sleep
- Affect eating habits
- Reduce energy
- Affect mood and concentration

Over time, it can contribute to long-term health problems.

Why Daily Habits Matter More Than Occasional Effort

Many people try to improve their health through short periods of effort.

They may eat well for a few days or exercise for a short time.

But health is shaped by what you do regularly.

Daily habits have a cumulative effect.

Simple routines such as:

- Going to bed at a consistent time
- Eating at regular intervals

- Taking breaks during the day
- Making time for relaxation

can make a meaningful difference over time.

The Connection Between Sleep, Stress, and Physical Health

Sleep and stress are closely connected.

Poor sleep can increase stress.

Stress can make it difficult to sleep.

This creates a cycle that can be difficult to break.

In addition:

- Stress may lead to unhealthy eating
- Poor sleep may reduce motivation for activity
- Both can affect blood pressure, weight, and blood sugar

Understanding this connection helps you address these issues more effectively.

How Irregular Routines Affect Your Health

An irregular daily pattern can disrupt the body's natural rhythm.

Examples include:

- Late-night schedules
- Irregular meal times

- Excessive screen time
- Lack of rest

These patterns can affect:

- Sleep quality
- Energy levels
- Mental clarity
- Overall well-being

Consistency in daily routine supports better health.

Creating a Healthier Daily Rhythm

Improving sleep and reducing stress do not require complex solutions.

Simple steps can help:

- Maintaining a regular sleep schedule
- Creating a calm environment before bedtime
- Taking short breaks during the day
- Practicing relaxation techniques
- Setting realistic daily expectations

Small changes, when practiced consistently, can lead to meaningful improvements.

Chronic Stress and Disease

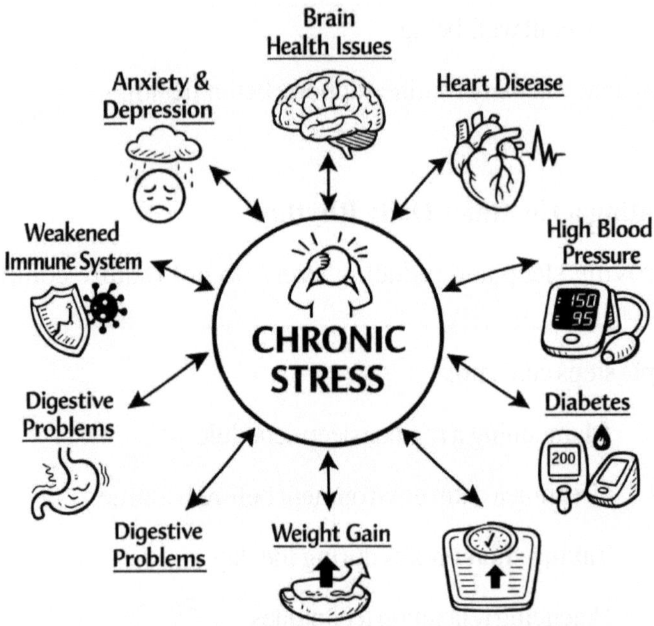

Chronic stress has harmful effects on the whole body.

Chapter Summary

- Sleep and stress have a strong impact on overall health.
- Poor sleep and chronic stress can affect many body systems.
- Daily habits influence health more than occasional effort.
- Sleep and stress are closely connected.
- Simple, consistent routines can improve well-being.

Action Plan

- Review your current sleep pattern.
- Aim for a consistent sleep schedule.
- Identify sources of stress in your daily life.
- Take one small step to reduce stress.
- Begin building a simple, stable daily routine.

Bridge to Chapter 12

Healthy habits are powerful, but they are not always enough on their own.

There are times when medical treatment plays an important role in protecting health.

Understanding how and when to use medicines wisely is essential.

Let us explore that next.

Chapter 12

When Medicines Help: Why Good Treatment and Good Habits Work Best Together

Many people feel a quiet resistance when the topic of medicines comes up.

It is a very human reaction.

No one wants to depend on medication. Many hope that with better diet, more exercise, and improved habits, medicines can be avoided altogether.

In some situations, that is possible.

But not always.

Understanding when medicines are helpful, and how they fit into the larger picture of health, is very important.

Why Healthy Living Alone Is Not Always Enough

Health is influenced by many factors.

Some are within your control:

- What you eat
- How much you move
- How well you sleep
- How you manage stress

But some factors are not fully within your control:

- Genetics
- Age-related changes
- The severity of a condition

For example:

- Some people develop high blood pressure despite a healthy lifestyle
- Blood sugar may remain elevated even with careful diet
- Cholesterol levels may be influenced by family history

In these situations, medicines may be necessary to protect the body.

Why Medicines Often Protect You from Serious Complications

Medicines are often prescribed not just to improve numbers, but to prevent future harm.

For example:

- Controlling blood pressure reduces the risk of stroke and heart disease
- Managing blood sugar helps protect the eyes, kidneys, and nerves
- Lowering cholesterol reduces the risk of heart attack

These benefits are not always immediately visible.

But over time, they can be very significant.

Why Many People Hesitate to Start Medicines

It is very common to feel uncertain about starting medication.

Some common concerns include:

- Fear of side effects
- Concern about long-term use
- A desire to avoid dependency
- Hearing negative experiences from others

These concerns are understandable.

However, avoiding necessary treatment may allow the condition to worsen.

The Risks of Stopping or Using Medicines Incorrectly

Another important issue is how medicines are used.

Some people:

- Stop medication when they start to feel better
- Skip doses
- Change doses without guidance
- Take medicines inconsistently

These patterns can reduce effectiveness and may even be harmful.

Many medicines need to be taken regularly to provide full benefit.

Why Medicines and Lifestyle Should Work Together

It is helpful to think of medicines and lifestyle as partners.

Not as alternatives.

Healthy habits can:

- Improve the effectiveness of medicines
- Reduce the need for higher doses
- Support better overall outcomes

In some cases, good lifestyle changes may allow reduction of medication over time.

But this should always be done carefully and under medical guidance.

Becoming a Confident and Informed Medicine User

Understanding your treatment is important.

You should know:

- Why a medicine has been prescribed
- What it is expected to do
- How and when to take it
- What side effects to watch for

This knowledge increases confidence and helps you use medicines more effectively.

It also improves communication with your doctor.

Chapter Summary

- Lifestyle is important, but it is not always sufficient on its own.
- Medicines can help prevent serious complications.
- Many people hesitate to start medicines due to understandable concerns.
- Incorrect use of medicines can reduce their benefit.
- The best outcomes often come from combining healthy habits with appropriate treatment.

Action Plan

- Reflect on your attitude toward medicines.
- Identify any concerns or misconceptions.
- Learn the purpose of each medicine you take.

- Take medicines as prescribed.
- Work with your doctor to balance lifestyle changes and treatment.

Bridge to Chapter 13

Even the best treatment works better when problems are identified early.

Many serious conditions develop quietly, without symptoms.

That is why prevention and regular checkups are so important.

Let us explore that next.

Chapter 13

Prevention and Checkups: The Quiet Protection Most People Undervalue

Most people seek medical care when something feels wrong.

That is natural. Pain, discomfort, or a worrying symptom brings attention immediately.

But some of the most important steps in protecting your health happen before anything feels wrong.

They happen quietly, through prevention and regular checkups.

Why Prevention Is One of the Wisest Health Decisions You Can Make

Prevention means taking steps to reduce the chance of disease before it develops or becomes serious.

It includes:

- Healthy daily habits
- Regular monitoring of important health indicators
- Early attention to small changes

These steps may seem simple.

But their long-term impact can be profound.

Prevention often avoids problems that would otherwise require more complex treatment later.

Why Feeling Well Does Not Always Mean Being Healthy

One of the most important realities in health is this:

You can feel well and still have a developing problem.

Conditions such as:

- High blood pressure
- High cholesterol
- Early diabetes

often do not cause noticeable symptoms in the beginning.

A person may feel normal while changes are taking place inside the body.

This is why relying only on how you feel is not enough.

The Role of Regular Checkups and Screening Tests

Regular medical checkups help identify problems early.

These may include:

- Blood pressure measurement
- Blood tests for sugar and cholesterol
- Weight and body measurements
- Age-appropriate screening tests

Early detection allows:

- Earlier treatment
- Better control
- Reduced risk of complications

Checkups are not only for those who are unwell. They are an important part of staying well.

Why Small Changes Should Not Be Ignored

Sometimes results show small or borderline changes.

It is easy to dismiss them.

But these early signs often represent the beginning of a trend.

Examples include:

- Slightly elevated blood pressure
- Mildly increased blood sugar
- Gradual weight gain

Addressing these early can prevent progression.

Small changes today can prevent larger problems tomorrow.

How Prevention Supports Peace of Mind

Prevention is not only about avoiding disease.

It also reduces uncertainty.

Knowing your health status can:

- Provide reassurance
- Reduce anxiety
- Help you plan and act wisely

Regular monitoring gives you a clearer picture of your health.

Why Prevention Saves Time, Effort, and Cost

Treating advanced disease often requires:

- More medications
- More frequent visits
- More complex care

Prevention often involves simpler steps.

It can:

- Reduce the need for intensive treatment
- Lower long-term healthcare costs
- Preserve quality of life

The benefits are both medical and practical.

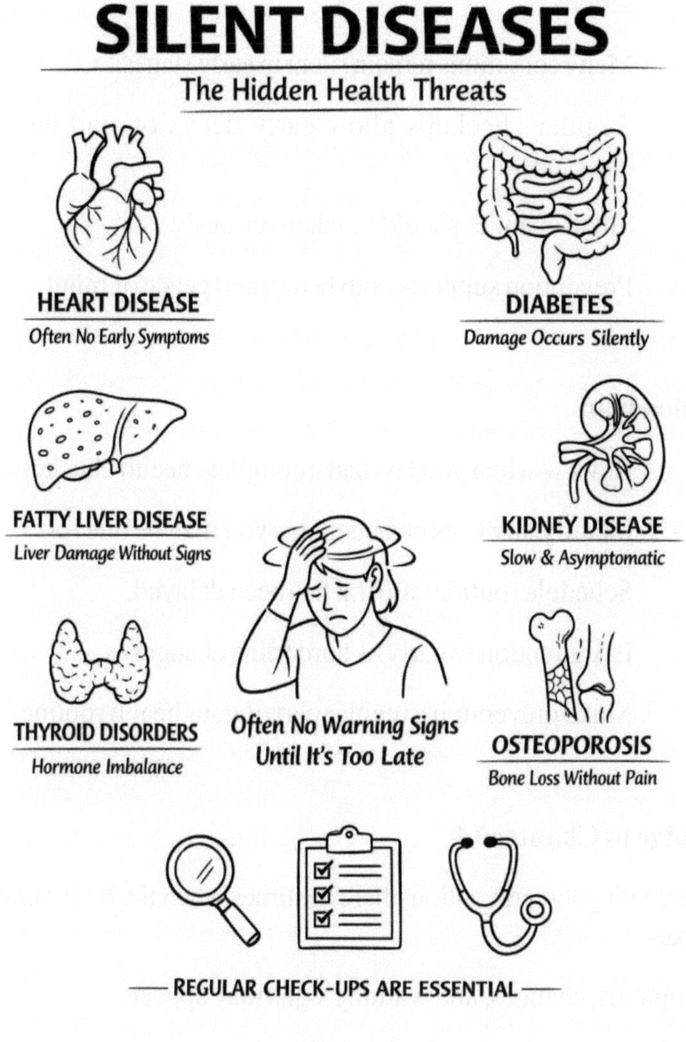
SILENT DISEASES
The Hidden Health Threats
HEART DISEASE
Often No Early Symptoms
DIABETES
Damage Occurs Silently
FATTY LIVER DISEASE
Liver Damage Without Signs
KIDNEY DISEASE
Slow & Asymptomatic
THYROID DISORDERS
Hormone Imbalance
Often No Warning Signs
Until It's Too Late
OSTEOPOROSIS
Bone Loss Without Pain
REGULAR CHECK-UPS ARE ESSENTIAL

Chapter Summary

- Prevention reduces the risk of disease before it becomes serious.
- Many conditions remain silent in early stages.
- Regular checkups allow early detection and better outcomes.
- Small changes should be taken seriously.
- Prevention supports both health and peace of mind.

Action Plan

- Review when you last had a complete health checkup.
- Identify any tests or screenings you may be due for.
- Schedule routine care if it has been delayed.
- Pay attention to early or borderline changes.
- Make prevention a regular part of your health routine.

Bridge to Chapter 14

Even with good prevention, there are times when the body sends signals.

Symptoms, changes, and warning signs may appear.

Recognizing these signals and responding appropriately is very important.

Let us explore that next.

Chapter 14

Do Not Ignore the Signals: Symptoms, Changes, and Warning Signs That Deserve Attention

The body has its own language.

It does not speak in words, but it communicates in other ways. A new discomfort. A change in energy. A pattern that was not there before. A symptom that lingers longer than expected.

These are messages.

Sometimes they are minor. Sometimes they are important.

The challenge is not to become fearful of every small change, but also not to ignore signals that deserve attention.

Learning this balance can protect your health in a very meaningful way.

Why People Often Delay Seeking Medical Attention

Many people notice changes in their body but do not act on them.

This is very common, and there are understandable reasons:

- Assuming the problem is minor
- Hoping it will go away on its own
- Being too busy
- Fear of what the diagnosis might be
- Gradually getting used to the symptom

At times, people normalize what they are experiencing.

What starts as a mild symptom slowly becomes "normal" for them.

This delay can sometimes allow a manageable problem to become more serious.

Why Early Warning Signs Are Often Subtle

Serious conditions do not always begin dramatically.

In many cases, the earliest signs are mild and easy to overlook.

Examples include:

- Unusual fatigue
- Reduced stamina
- Mild but persistent discomfort
- Changes in appetite or weight

- Sleep disturbances

Because these symptoms are not severe, they are often dismissed.

Paying attention to these early signs can help identify problems sooner.

The Danger of Accepting What Is Not Normal

It is easy to attribute many symptoms to aging or stress.

While some changes are natural, not everything should be accepted without question.

For example:

- Persistent fatigue is not always "just aging"
- Shortness of breath should not be ignored
- New or worsening pain deserves evaluation
- Unexplained weight change may signal an underlying issue

Accepting abnormal symptoms as normal can delay proper care.

When to Observe, When to Act, and When to Seek Urgent Care

Not every symptom requires immediate medical attention.

But it is important to develop a thoughtful approach.

- **Observation** is reasonable for minor, short-term symptoms
- **Timely consultation** is needed for symptoms that persist

or worsen

- **Urgent care** is required for severe or sudden symptoms

Symptoms that should never be ignored include:

- Chest discomfort
- Severe shortness of breath
- Sudden weakness or difficulty speaking
- Changes in consciousness

Knowing when to act is an important part of self-care.

Why Early Action Leads to Better Outcomes

When problems are addressed early:

- Treatment is often simpler
- Complications are less likely
- Recovery may be faster

When attention is delayed:

- Conditions may progress
- Treatment may become more complex
- Outcomes may be less favorable

Timely action can make a significant difference.

Listening to Your Body Without Becoming Anxious

Awareness is important, but so is balance.

It is not helpful to become overly worried about every small change.

The goal is:

- Awareness without fear
- Attention without overreaction
- Thoughtful action when needed

Over time, you will learn what is usual for you and what is not.

Chapter Summary

- The body communicates through symptoms and changes.
- Many people delay seeking care for understandable reasons.
- Early warning signs are often subtle.
- Not all symptoms should be accepted as normal.
- Timely attention can improve outcomes.
- Balanced awareness is more helpful than either neglect or excessive worry.

Action Plan

- Think about any symptoms or changes you may have been ignoring.

- Do not assume persistent changes are normal without evaluation.
- Seek medical advice for symptoms that continue or worsen.
- Learn to distinguish between minor issues and those needing attention.
- Practice awareness without unnecessary anxiety.

Bridge to Chapter 15

You now have a broad understanding of how health works.

The final step is to bring everything together.

How can you use this knowledge in a practical way?

How can this book, along with the rest of the series, guide you in protecting your health over time?

Let us explore that in the final chapter.

Chapter 15

One Person, Many Health Issues: How to Use This Series to Protect Your Health as a Whole

You have now reached the end of this book, but in many ways, this is where your real journey begins.

Over the past chapters, we have stepped back and looked at health from a wider and more thoughtful perspective. You have seen that health is not one single decision, one diagnosis, or one treatment. It is a combination of many factors working together over time.

You have also seen something even more important.

You are not a collection of separate problems.

You are one whole person.

This final chapter is about bringing everything together and showing you how to use this understanding in your daily life.

Why This Series Is Designed as a Connected Whole

Health is too important to be reduced to isolated pieces of information.

At the same time, it is also too complex to be fully explained in a single book.

That is why this series has been designed as a connected set of books.

Each book focuses on one topic so that it can be explained clearly and in enough depth. At the same time, all the books are connected by a common purpose.

This allows you to:

- Understand each condition more clearly
- See how different aspects of health relate to each other
- Apply knowledge in a more practical way

Why Diseases Are Discussed Separately, but Not Truly Separate

For clarity, we often talk about diseases one at a time.

We may say:

- "This is diabetes"
- "This is high blood pressure"
- "This is heart disease"

But in real life, these conditions are not isolated.

They are closely linked.

For example:

- Weight can influence blood sugar and blood pressure
- Blood pressure can affect the heart, brain, and kidneys
- Cholesterol affects blood vessels throughout the body

Understanding this connection helps you see the bigger picture.

How One Book Strengthens Your Understanding of Another

Each book in this series supports the others.

When you read about one condition, you begin to recognize how it connects with others.

For example:

- Understanding weight can help you understand diabetes
- Learning about blood pressure can help you understand heart health
- Improving sleep and lifestyle can influence multiple conditions

This interconnected understanding makes your knowledge more useful.

Why Reading Across the Series Makes You More Prepared

When you understand your health more clearly:

- You ask better questions
- You make more thoughtful decisions

- You follow treatment plans more effectively

You are no longer dependent only on brief conversations.

You become an active participant in your own care.

This leads to:

- Better communication with your doctor
- Greater confidence
- Better long-term outcomes

How to Choose What to Read Next

You do not need to read everything at once.

Start with what is most relevant to you.

Consider:

- Your current health conditions
- Your risk factors
- Your family history
- Your lifestyle

For example:

- If you are concerned about weight, start there
- If you have high blood pressure, focus on that
- If you want a broader understanding, revisit this book

Over time, you can expand your reading.

Becoming an Active Partner in Your Own Health

The purpose of this series is not only to provide information.

It is to help you become:

- More aware
- More informed
- More confident
- More involved in your own care

Health decisions do not happen only in a doctor's office.

They happen every day, through your choices and your understanding.

When you take an active role:

- You protect your health more effectively
- You reduce confusion and fear
- You improve your quality of life

Chapter Summary

- Health is made up of many interconnected factors.
- Diseases are discussed separately for clarity but are connected in reality.
- The books in this series are designed to work together.
- Reading across the series improves understanding and decision-making.

Better Health with Dr Das Series

How it Will Help You

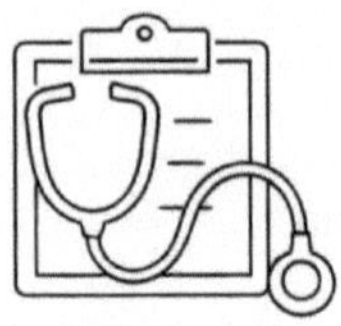

Medical Advice

Expert Tips on Health & Wellness

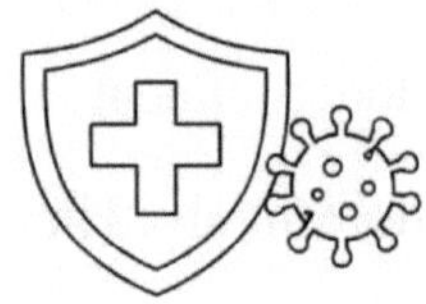

Disease Prevention

Learn to Prevent Illnesses

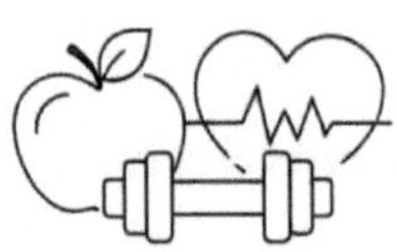

Healthy Lifestyle

Nutrition & Fitness Guidance

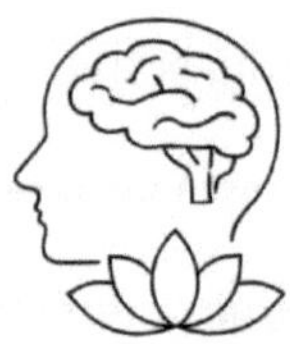

Mental Wellbeing

Stress Management & Mindfidness

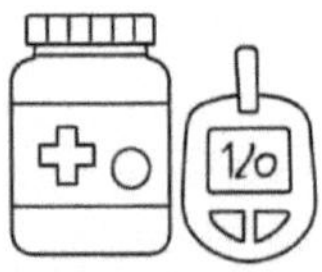

Chronic Conditions

Managing Long-Term Illnesses

Q&A Sessions

Your Health Questions Answered

- Becoming an informed and active participant is essential for long-term health.

Action Plan

- Identify the health areas most relevant to you right now.
- Choose one or two books in this series to read next.
- Use this anchor book as your foundation.
- Take a more active role in understanding your health.
- Commit to ongoing learning and steady improvement.

Final Thought

Better health is not created in one moment.

It is built slowly.

It is built through:

- Understanding
- Awareness
- Daily choices
- Consistent effort

This book has given you a foundation.

What you do next will shape your future.

Better health is not far away.

Thank You and Please Review the Book

Thank you for taking the time to read this book. I sincerely hope it has helped you understand your health a little more clearly and has given you practical, everyday steps you can follow with confidence. If you found this book helpful, **I would truly appreciate it if you could leave a brief and honest review**. Even a few lines sharing your experience can make a meaningful difference. Your feedback helps other readers find reliable, trustworthy health information and supports them in making better decisions for themselves and their families.

Warm regards,

Dr Prabhat Das

Continue your Healthcare Journey

Good health is a journey, not a single step. It is not achieved in one day or with one book. That is why I created the **"Better Health with Dr Das"** series, with each book addressing a different common condition. If you would like easy, practical guidance on other everyday health concerns, you may wish to explore the rest of books in this series.

Books in this series:

- **Better Health Starts Here:** A Doctor's Guide to Staying **Healthy After 40**
- A Doctor's Easy Guide to Understanding & Managing **OBESITY.**
- A Doctor's Easy Guide to Understanding & Managing **HIGH BLOOD PRESSURE.**
- Doctor, **What DIET** Is Best for Me?
- Doctor, Why Can't I **Lose Weight?**

  (a Doctor's Guide to safe & Sustainable Weight Loss)
- A Doctor's Easy Guide to **GLP-1 for Obesity**

- A Doctor's Guide to **Living Well With DIABETES**
- A Doctor's Guide to Understanding & Managing **HIGH CHOLESTEROL**
- A Doctor's Guide to Understanding & Managing **THYROID DISEASES**
- Several other books on other common health conditions are coming soon…

9 781971 672236

Printed by Libri Plureos GmbH in Hamburg, Germany